Four Secrets of Healthy Families

CHARLES T. KUNTZLEMAN

POCKET GUIDES
Tyndale House Publishers, Inc.
Wheaton, Illinois

Adapted from *The Well Family Book,* copyright 1985 by Here's Life
Publishers, Inc. Used by permission.

First printing, November 1988
Library of Congress Catalog Card Number 88-51237
ISBN 0-8423-0831-8

CONTENTS

PREFACE

This book is based on thirteen years of extensive research on Feelin' Good, a cardiovascular fitness program for kindergarten through ninth grade. Feelin' Good teaches public and private school children how to assume responsibility for their own health through exercise, food, weight, stress management, and saying no to smoking and drugs. I call this responsibility the fourth R in education.

The program started in 1973. It was field-tested by children, teachers, and parents in the San Diego Unified School District. In 1976, the program was introduced to hundreds of YMCAs across the United States as part of the nationwide cardiovascular health program. In 1980, a \$481,219 grant from the W. K. Kellogg Foundation allowed researchers to evaluate the program's effectiveness in all Jackson County, Michigan, schools. The conclusion: Strategies employed in Feelin' Good teach children how to reduce their risk of cardiovascular disease and body fat, improve their fitness level, increase their activity patterns, improve the quality of their eating, and enhance their self-esteem.

During this same time, I developed and helped evaluate adult health, fitness, and wellness programs for the YMCA of the USA, Campbell's Soups, Phillips Petroleum, Ross Laboratories, Rodale Press, and other corporations, hospitals, schools, and universities. I also developed the Living Well program—a nationwide health enhancement program for corporations and hospitals.

In my work with children and adults, I realized that wellness starts in the home. Health patterns and behaviors established in childhood have a profound effect on adults' exercise, eating, stress, weight, and addiction habits, and, therefore, upon their current health and vitality.

While many of the ideas presented here are based on experiences and ideas used in Feelin' Good, you'll also find experiences and activities that my wife, Beth, and I have used with our five children—ages seventeen to twenty-five. These concepts are reinforced with further views from participants in our health and well-being classes in Jackson County, Michigan, and other fitness professionals around the world.

Now, before you think that I have discovered the secret of raising kids and making them healthy, wealthy, and wise, please be assured that the same things do not work with every child. We've had our share of successes and, certainly, our share of failures. My advice is to try the strategies—I think you'll find them effective. But be flexible enough to change and modify if things don't seem to work as outlined.

So let's start a journey—a journey that can be exciting and, yes, at times, frustrating, but a journey that with God's help will make your family feel better. It will enable you and yours to enjoy some of this life's promised fulfillments.

Taking Stock: How Healthy Is Your Family

Good family health. That's a dream of us all. We want our children, spouses, and selves to live well, free from runny noses, allergies, tummy aches, and athlete's foot. Yet we can deal with these things, and scores of books tell us how.

Heart attacks, cancer, diabetes, strokes, and other catastrophic diseases are another story. These strike fear and terror in our hearts. These are diseases that ruin our family's quality of life. These are afflictions that take parents from children. Modern day plagues that kill or maim all family members. Unfortunately, not many books give parents guidelines on how to help their family avoid these dreaded diseases.

As a specialist in exercise, fitness, and wellness, I am dismayed at the number of people struck by these afflictions. Dismayed because more than 50 percent of these deaths and ailments could be prevented by a change in living habits. The seeds for these diseases are planted in childhood, nurtured during adolescence, and come to full bloom in adulthood.

FIVE REASONS KIDS DON'T LEARN HEALTH

As parents, we promote the spiritual, mental, and social health of our children to prepare them for life's battles, battles they will encounter as adults. We expend a tremendous amount of energy to help them have successful relationships. We try to serve as good role models. We help fine-tune our children's intellectual abilities. That is all good and as it should be.

Unfortunately, when it comes to their skills and abilities to fight heart disease, cancer, diabetes, cirrhosis, emphysema, asthma, arthritis, ulcers, depression, obesity, and fatigue, we fall short. We focus on the here-and-now diseases — such non-life-threatening ailments as colds, stomachaches, and headaches. We fail to give our children a fighting chance to ward off the degenerative and debilitating diseases that will rob them and their future families of much joy and happiness. Why is this so?

1. *Ignorance.* I believe that one reason we don't give our children a chance to fight degenerative disease is that we don't know what kind of family activities to get involved in to encourage good future health.

2. *A faulty definition of health*. We view health as the absence of disease. Most of us take our health for granted (although we fear being sick) until it is almost too late. We decide to get well *after* we are too sick to function properly. Then we seek relief or professional help and expect a quick cure —Valium to calm down, Dexatrim to lose weight, nitroglycerin to prevent chest pain. These quick "cures" plus

billions of dollars spent mask our real problem—our life-style. We are not willing to change our way of living and thinking to improve our health and vitality. So we try to repair our health *after* we lose it.

3. *Our culture.* We often allow our culture to dictate our living habits, despite the fact that we "know better" and have been deluged with facts and figures on the dangers of smoking, too rich a diet, alcohol, and sedentary living.

4. *Habits.* Our current life-style and habits are convenient, easy, and pleasurable. My own experience with people validates a recent poll conducted at Pennsylvania State University on women between the ages of twenty and fifty-nine. The study revealed that 58 percent of American women haven't changed their eating habits because the emphasis of food selection is based on taste, not nutrition.

5. *Faulty assumptions.* We assume our children cannot make decisions for themselves. We teach them passivity in health care. We tell them when to take their shots and medicine. Mom, Dad, and the doctor talk while Billy and Suzie stare at the wall or finger a pencil on the desk.

Yet a recent study showed that kids actually heal faster if they are encouraged to help themselves. Studies conducted at the University of Wisconsin Medical School showed that two- to twelve-year-olds recovered quicker from second- and third-degree burns if they cleaned and dressed their own wounds.[1] Extensive studies on asthmatics showed similar results. Children who were taught what sets off an at-

The State of Health in the U.S.

Adults

- 70% drink alcoholic beverages
- 30% smoke cigarettes
- 53% *never* wear seat belts in a car
- 64% do not get enough exercise (24% never exercise)
- 35% or more are overweight
- 50%-80% take a prescription drug every other day

Children

- 98% have at least one heart disease risk factor (high cholesterol, high blood pressure, obesity, etc.); 13 percent have five or more risk factors
- 20%-25% carry too much body fat
- 28% rarely visit a doctor
- 40% *never* wear seat belts in a car
- 75% have diets that include too much fat[2]

tack, how to recognize early warning signs, when and how to medicate, and how drugs work had fewer emergency room visits and missed fewer school days.[3]

HEALTH: WORTH THE EFFORT

One of God's greatest gifts to us is the organization of this universe. Attempt to defy the law of gravity by jumping off a ten-story building and you will be killed. Swim in icy water for any length of time and you'll freeze to death. You simply cannot go against God's laws of the universe.

The same applies to your body health. Go against God's laws of health, and your vitality and vigor will be affected. And your life may be cut short.

In the 1960s and 1970s, Drs. Nedra Belloc and Lester Breslow of UCLA studied 6,928 adults in Alameda County, California. They discovered that people who adopted six or seven basic health habits lived seven (women) to eleven (men) years longer than those people who practiced three or less of these habits.

Interestingly, these habits were not complicated. They were things your grandmother probably told you to do: (1) Get regular, moderate exercise; (2) eat breakfast every day; (3) have regular meals with no snacks in between; (4) maintain normal weight; (5) get seven to eight hours of sleep a night; (6) do not smoke; (7) drink alcohol in small amounts (one to two ounces a day) or not at all.[4]

You may be thinking, *What about the guy on my street who was overweight, ate fatty meals, smoked big black cigars, drank whiskey, and died at the age of 92?*

This person was an exception. He also probably would have lived even longer if he'd had a healthier life-style. The latest research suggests that we inherit our parents' (and their parents') potential for longevity.[5] But our circumstances and daily choices may chop months or years from those God has allotted to us.

The allotted number of years is an important

concept. It explains differences in longevity despite dissimilar health behaviors. One person may be granted a possible lifespan of 100 years and another, 80. The potential 100-year-old may adopt an unhealthy life-style and die at the age of 81. The potential 80-year-old may follow so-called well behaviors and live to be 75. The unhealthy person lost one-fifth of his allotted years; the healthy person, one-sixteenth. The former is a travesty of a precious gift.

But health is not necessarily longevity—adding years to your life. It *is* adding life to your years. How many times have you come home from the office and, after working all day, can't seem to do anything more? The kids want to play, but you're too tired. Your spouse wants to go shopping, but you want to sit. The zing is gone. Aging? Probably not. It's more likely a lack of fitness.

Let's take the examples above. The person who reached 75 years based on a possible God-given 80 undoubtedly had a life of vigor, energy, and relatively good health. The 81-year-old who had the potential for 100 years probably was plagued with chronic bronchitis or emphysema from smoking, sluggish bowels from a poor diet, low back pain from obesity, headaches from unresolved stress, and a lack of energy because of poor fitness. So the abusive life-style cuts deep. It robs a person of longevity and *joie de vivre*.

I don't mean to imply that if you're fit you won't have any health problems. Most of us carry within us the microbes that cause influenza, tuberculosis, staph infections, and other illnesses—including the common cold. When we get into a family or office argument, stay up late, eat poorly, or overdo work or some chemical, our resistance is lowered. When that happens repeatedly, these microbes can take hold. But improved health habits and well-being help you roll with the blows you receive in life, reduce your chances for or severity of disease, keep the microbes in check, and help you experience the wholeness God intended for you and your family.

A CHECK-UP ON FAMILY HEALTH

Taking stock of family health is important. Don't deceive yourself into thinking all is well. Most Americans think their health is average. Sadly, to be average in America means you are unhealthy. Consider that one in two of us will die of heart disease, one in four will develop cancer, nine out of ten will have neck or back pain, and almost four out of ten will be overweight.

Tragically, these problems start in childhood. The behaviors and habits developed now in your children will carry over into adulthood. The heart attack at fifty started at age five. The obesity of middle age began during the first few years of life.

Table 1 has three checklists, one for each of the three areas of health I will talk about in this guide—fitness, food, and weight. The checklists will help you define the area of health that you or members of your family should work on.

Once you've identified your major area of concern, have your children and spouse take the test as well. You will need to read or answer the questions for children under nine or ten years of age.

To get started, look over Table 1. After each entry, you'll find six statements. Read each one carefully, and circle the number on the left that best describes your level of achievement. Then check the box on the right that indicates your level of satisfaction. Are you pleased with your level of achievement, or do you think you need to improve? If you scored poorly in a given area, yet you are really satisfied to stay at that level, admit it. Remember, this is only for you and your family. No one has to know what you think of yourself except you.

Next, discuss with your spouse the questions in Table 2. If you checked all ten as yes, congratulations! Wherever there is a no, you and your spouse need to look at techniques to improve your responses.

In addition to these questions, ask each other, "Are we willing, with God's help, to do what it takes to improve our family's health? Are we willing to affirm each other's efforts and those of our children?" If the answer is no, close this book now. If it is yes, read on.

MOVING INTO ACTION

1. *Admit you have a problem*. This is perhaps one of the most difficult steps in any plan of action. It's also the most necessary. Unless you

TABLE 1
PERSONAL HEALTH CHECKLIST
Enjoying Exercise (Fitness)

Level of Achievement							Level of Satisfaction		
Low				High			OK	Needs Improvement	Could be Improved but Not a Concern at This Time
1	2	3	4	5	a.	I bike, swim, run, or walk for at least 30 minutes, three or more times a week.	☐	☐	☐
1	2	3	4	5	b.	Whenever possible, I walk or ride a bike instead of using cars, elevators, escalators.	☐	☐	☐
1	2	3	4	5	c.	I do some form of stretching several times per week.	☐		☐
1	2	3	4	5	d.	I work on muscle fitness three times a week.	☐	☐	☐☐☐
1	2	3	4	5	e.	It is fun for me to be physically active.	☐	☐	
1	2	3	4	5	f.	I try to learn one new sport every two years.	☐	☐	

Eating Well (Food)

Level of Achievement		Level of Satisfaction		
Low 1 2 3 4 5 High		OK	Needs Improvement	Could be Improved but Not a Concern at This Time
1 2 3 4 5	a. I eat a balanced diet and enjoy a variety of fresh, natural foods.	☐	☐	☐
1 2 3 4 5	b. I try to eat foods with little added sugar, salt, and/or saturated fat.	☐	☐	☐
1 2 3 4 5	c. I take time to relax and enjoy my meals. I also eat my food in one location (at a table).	☐	☐	☐
1 2 3 4 5	d. I consume very little coffee, colas, or other foods high in caffeine.	☐	☐	☐
1 2 3 4 5	e. I eat three well-balanced meals a day—breakfast, lunch, and dinner.	☐	☐	☐
1 2 3 4 5	f. I do not eat in fast food restaurants more than one to two times a month. When I do, I'm careful to select the most healthful foods.	☐	☐	☐

Staying Slim (Weight)

Level of Achievement (Low — High)		Level of Satisfaction
		OK Needs Improvement Could be Improved but Not a Concern at This Time
1 2 3 4 5	a. I bike, swim, run, or walk for at least 30 minutes, three or more times a week.	☐ ☐
1 2 3 4 5	b. I eat foods high in nutrients and low in calories three times a day.	☐ ☐
1 2 3 4 5	c. I don't eat when I'm bored or under pressure.	☐ ☐ ☐ ☐
1 2 3 4 5	d. I cannot pinch more than an inch of fat on my body.	
1 2 3 4 5	e. I am satisfied with the way my body looks.	☐ ☐ ☐ ☐
1 2 3 4 5	f. I do not worship my body by attempting to be excessively slim or exceptionally well-built.	

TABLE 2

FAMILY HEALTH CHECKLIST

	Circle One
As parents, we actively, constructively, and consistently:	
a. Engage in and provide opportunities for our family to get regular physical exercise.	YES NO
b. Engage in and provide opportunities for our family to walk or ride bikes, rather than use motorized vehicles.	YES NO
c. Provide nutritious meals that are low in salt, fat, cholesterol, and sugar.	YES NO
d. Provide snacks that are healthy and nutritious, i.e. fruit, vegetables, fruit juices, whole grain breads, etc.	YES NO
e. Reinforce positive pictures of the children's bodies and avoid put-downs such as, "You're fat" or "You've put weight on lately, haven't you?"	YES NO
f. Support our spouse's or children's attempts to control their weight through proper exercise and appropriate eating habits.	YES NO

admit that you or your family have a problem, you never will solve it.

Look at Table 1 and pinpoint those areas where you feel you need improvement. That's where you need to start in your quest for a healthier life. Each of the following chapters corresponds to one of these areas of health. Just remember, you can't attack everything at once. Pick one area and go from there.

2. *Focus on the reasons.* Once you admit that a certain area presents a problem to you and decide to do something about it, try to be specific. For example, let's say you are not satisfied with your eating patterns and you decide to change the way you eat. You select item *c* under "Eating Well" as an area that needs improvement because you do not take time to relax and enjoy your meals. You eat your food on the run or in front of the television.

Taking stock of that problem involves a closer look at mealtime. Why don't you take the time to relax and enjoy meals? What causes you to hurry? How much time is actually spent at the table? What sort of activities are taking place while you are eating? Answering these questions will help you pinpoint why this is a problem. The key to this step is determining how it developed into a problem. Once you see the causes, you can devise ways to minimize it.

3. *Work together as a family.* It's much better if everyone is pushing for a common goal. That is, all are attempting to eat better, lose weight, or exercise more.

Personally, I find it easiest to start off with a new habit myself, or my wife, Beth, will initiate the idea. We'll talk about it and see if the other wants to go along. Then we will try it for a period of time. After observing us, some of the children decide to participate, without direct encouragement. Other times, they need to be coaxed.

Sometimes family members never join in on an activity, however, and you need to respect their right to pass. Personal example, excitement for a habit, reward for involvement, the majority of the family participating, and making health habits fun are better motivators than nagging.

4. *Expect change to take time!* You never graduate from the school of health and well-being. It is a lifelong, dynamic process. You make commitments, evaluate changes, and then decide to keep, change, or modify as you experience new healthful techniques.

Here is a summary of my family's commitment to building better physical health, with an emphasis on some of my personal decisions.

AGE HEALTH STAGE
21 Married.
22 Debbie born.
    Cut back on salting my food.
23 John born.
27 Reduced personal sugar consumption.
    Thomas born.
29 Reduced children's salt intake.
    Reduced saturated fat/cholesterol in my diet.
    Started taking vitamins.
    Rebecca born.

31 Increased my distance running to four
    to five miles a day (five days a week).
32 Developed and practiced neuromus-
    cular relaxation techniques.
    First wife died.   •
    Had children reduce their saturated
    fat/cholesterol intake.
33 Personally decided not to use medi-
    cine of any type.
34 Remarried.
    Increased long-distance mileage to six
    miles (five to six days a week).
    Set up reward system for children to
    exercise.
    Reduced children's sugar intake.
    Cut way back on processed foods.
35 Supplemented family diet with
    vitamins.
35 Took the television out of the house.
37 Dropped neuromuscular techniques
    and picked up relaxation response
    and body-scanning techniques.
    Cut back on red meat consumption
    for all family members.
38 Decided to use medicine for allergies.
39 Started mineral supplementation for
    family and personal use.
    Flirted with vegetarianism.
40 Brought television back into the
    house.
    Returned to eating meat one to two
    days each week.
41 Gave up fruit during ragweed season
    to reduce allergies.
42 Two daughters highly allergic, so rota-
    tional diets established for them.
44 Created a family fitness room in the
    basement.

As you can see, we made health changes when we were ready. Also, we sometimes made changes when we reevaluated previous decisions. For example, I went off all medication, yet my allergies plagued me, so I resorted to over-the-counter medication to help me through extremely difficult times. The television was taken out of the house for a period of at least three years. We brought it back in because some family members like to watch certain shows. (Besides, the children lobbied for it.)

The point is, building personal health is not something you do overnight. It's a maturation process. You gradually understand or realize what does and does not work for you. My personal changes and those of the family came slowly; yours must too.

The next chapters will show you how to start making the changes that will enable your family to enjoy the benefits of good health.

CHAPTER 2

Making Family Fitness Fun!

What is physical fitness? It is the capacity of your body to meet the demands of your day (or any unexpected emergencies) without undue fatigue. The demands might include shoveling snow for thirty minutes, climbing thirty flights of stairs, putting shrubbery in the yard, or playing basketball with the kids.

To meet these demands without fear of over-exertion, you and your family must develop four major components of physical fitness: cardiovascular endurance, proper body composition/weight ratio, muscle fitness, and flexibility. Let's look at each of these.

CARDIOVASCULAR ENDURANCE

Cardiovascular endurance is the fitness of your heart, blood, blood vessels, and lungs. A high level of cardiovascular endurance means that your body can transport and use oxygen efficiently.

Improving your cardiovascular endurance definitely will improve your stamina and energy level. In fact, without a good level of cardiovascular endurance, you almost always will feel below par—too tired to do family chores or be involved in family fun.

Good cardiovascular endurance seems to play a role in reducing your risk of heart disease, as well. In 1976, Dr. Kenneth H. Cooper and some of his associates presented research that compared cardiovascular risk factors and fitness levels of 3,000 men who had come to the Cooper Clinic between 1971 and 1974. The study results showed striking consistencies. Men who were in very poor and poor condition showed uniformly poor results. Predictably, their cholesterol, triglyceride, glucose, uric acid, systolic and diastolic pressures, and body fat values were substantially poorer than the men who had good to excellent cardiovascular endurance.[1]

Intrigued by Dr. Cooper's research, we did a similar study with children ages seven to twelve. Our results were almost identical. As the children's cardiovascular endurance levels increased, their cardiovascular risk factors decreased significantly.

Improved physical fitness is important for children, especially since researchers believe that heart disease begins in childhood. Fat deposits are found early in life. By age three, nearly *all* American children have some fat deposits on the inner surface of the aorta (the body's largest artery). These deposits increase rapidly after age eight, and at age fifteen have affected 15 percent of the aorta's surface. Yet children in primitive countries do not have

Health Hazard: Heart Disease

The major killer and crippler in the U.S. is heart disease. Almost 50 percent of all Americans die of heart attacks, strokes, and kidney failure. Many are stricken in the prime of life (thirty-five to fifty-five years of age). The 50 percent who survive the first heart attack have a life expectancy of five to seven years.[2]

Heart disease takes many forms. Degenerative coronary artery disease is the most insidious; the heart's blood vessels degenerate due to a build-up of fats on their lining. The build-up, if uncontrolled for a period of time, eventually will block blood circulation with the formation of a clot, called a thrombosis. This blockage may occur anywhere in the body. In the heart it is called a heart attack; in the brain, a stroke; in the kidney, it is called kidney failure.

Science is making strides in treating heart disease, but the key is in preventing or slowing it. Heart disease appears to be caused by our lifestyle. Fifty percent of all heart attacks and strokes could be prevented by:[3]

- stopping smoking
- reducing elevated blood pressure
- reducing blood fats (blood cholesterol)
- modifying the diet (reducing cholesterol, saturated fat, salt, and sugar consumption)
- increasing physical fitness
- reducing weight and body fat
- dealing positively with stress

these fatty deposits. It seems, therefore, that these blood vessel changes are due to habits. Research we conducted on school-aged children in our county supports that view, since:

- 41% had cholesterols considered to be too high
- 29% had elevated triglycerides
- 12% had low levels of HDLs (high levels are a good sign)
- 15% had excessively high systolic blood pressures
- 28% had diastolic blood pressures that were too high

Exercise is also important for the heart health of adults. Since the early 1950s, numerous studies have been conducted to determine the effects of exercise on a person's chance of having a heart attack. The evidence is almost overwhelming. Active people have only about one-half the chance of having a heart attack as inactive people. Furthermore, if an active person has a heart attack, his survival chances are two to five times greater than the inactive person.

THE BENEFITS OF EXERCISE

Why is this so? Dr. Samuel Fox, professor of cardiology at Georgetown University in Washington, D.C., and Dr. William Haskell, associate professor at Stanford University in Palo Alto, California, have presented several possible reasons. According to these experts, exercise may:[4]

1. Increase the number and size of your blood vessels (causing better and more efficient circulation).

2. Increase the elasticity of blood vessels (less likelihood of breaking under pressure).

3. Increase the efficiency of exercising muscles and blood circulation (muscles and blood are better able to pick up, carry and use oxygen).

4. Increase the efficiency of the heart (able to pump more blood with fewer beats – better able to meet emergencies).

5. Increase tolerance to stress and give you more joy of living (so you will be less likely to be caught in the stress/pressure syndrome).

6. Decrease clot formation (less chance of blood clot forming and blocking blood flow to the heart muscle).

7. Decrease triglyceride and cholesterol levels (less likelihood of fats being deposited on the lining of the arteries).

8. Decrease blood sugar (reduce chances of blood sugar being changed to triglycerides).

9. Decrease obesity and high blood pressure (most people who are obese and have high blood pressure are more prone to heart disease).

10. Decrease hormone production (too much adrenaline can cause problems for the arteries).

Good cardiovascular endurance also has been shown to help people relieve headaches, reduce anxiety, lift people from depression, and stimulate creativity and confidence.

My daughter, Deb, is a case in point. Ten

years ago, at the age of fifteen, she started to run. Two years later, during an enjoyable father and daughter run, I said, "Deb, when you were fifteen you seemed more moody. If things didn't go your way, you'd get real quiet and sulk. Maybe even go out in the middle of the yard and sit for an hour or so. You don't do that any more. How come?"

"Oh, that's easy," she said. "My running changed all that. Maybe I'm more mature, too, but I noticed that about six months after I started running, I lost some of my tension and anger. It relaxed me."

That reinforced my opinion of the value of exercise. It said more than all the research studies I've read on the mental benefits of exercise.

Cardiovascular exercise is not a panacea, but the evidence is clear. Good cardiovascular endurance benefits your heart, mind, and energy levels. And cardiovascular endurance is improved with exercises such as walking, running, biking, swimming, cross-country skiing, rowing, and aerobics.

BODY COMPOSITION/WEIGHT RATIO
We will discuss this aspect of physical fitness in greater detail in chapter 4.

MUSCULAR FITNESS
Muscle fitness refers to the strength, endurance, and appearance of the various muscles of the body. A reasonable degree of muscle

strength is needed for moving and lifting heavy objects—everything from pianos to groceries.

From a health perspective, muscle fitness is necessary to avoid low back pain. In a study of 3,000 back pain patients at Columbia Presbyterian Medical Center, Al Melleby, retired director for the YMCA's Healthy Back Program, found that 83 percent of the back problems were of muscle origin.[5]

According to experts, our sedentary life heads us into back trouble. A lack of physical activity causes abdominal muscles to weaken and sag. In addition, we accumulate too much fat around our waists. To compensate for the sagging waistline, we arch our backs. Consequently, the pelvis tips forward. Our derriere sticks out. The last joints of the spine require a lot of muscle to hold them up. Eventually, the muscles in the lower back tire of carrying the load and they ache a bit. Most backaches with children are due to this poor posture or weak abdominal muscles.

With adults, the low backache syndrome starts with the same problems—weak muscles and too much fat. That is then aggravated by day to day tensions, which make the back muscles contract. When the muscles contract beyond a certain point, significant back pain occurs.

FLEXIBILITY
Flexibility is the range of motion possible at each of your joints. It is important for your good health because it helps prevent muscle pulls

Health Hazard: Headaches

Ninety percent of the population suffers from headaches sometime in their lives, 20 percent of which need treatment. Most headache sufferers are women between the ages of fourteen and forty-five. Dr. Harold G. Wolff, a pioneer student of headaches, notes that 95 percent of all headaches are caused by what he calls biological reprimands.[6] These reprimands tell you that something in your body is off balance. Your body makes adjustments to compensate for this lack of balance. These adjustments include tightened muscles and expanded blood vessels in the head and neck. The muscles and blood vessels then press upon and irritate neighboring tissues. In short, you get a headache.

The causes of headaches are endless and, unfortunately, different for practically everyone. Contributing factors include too much of the following: alcohol; chemicals in food, air, or water; light or glare that causes squinting; caffeine; pain-killing drugs; stress and tension; anger and frustration; and repressed anxiety. Headaches also may be caused by hunger, the lack of oxygen in high altitudes, and a very low barometric pressure. Preventing headaches is best done by practicing stress management techniques, exercising regularly, eating a proper diet, and avoiding alcohol, caffeine, drugs, and tobacco.

and strains. Improved flexibility results in fewer injuries and more freedom of movement. A lack of flexibility can contribute to low back pain and those maddening muscle and joint injuries that occur when you attempt to reach for an object underneath a desk or on top of a shelf.

Generally, flexibility is not a problem with children. The loss of flexibility starts during the teenage years and becomes obvious at about age thirty-five.

There is no such thing as a flexible person; there are only people with flexible joints. To improve your overall flexibility, you must work on each part of your body. Exercises best for this are those of the slow stretch nature.

There you have it! To be physically fit you must work on the four essentials of fitness — cardiovascular endurance, body composition/weight ratio, muscular fitness, and flexibility. Neglect of any essential element may cause injury, an imbalance in physical appearance, or lack of the potential benefits outlined here.

Let's move on to find out how you can be fit for life.

HOW TO HAVE A HEALTHY HEART
The amount of heart exercise you need depends upon your personal goals. Physiologists talk about the intensity (how hard), duration (how long), and frequency (how often) of exercise. They also recognize the interaction between intensity, duration, and frequency. That interaction creates a fourth factor — total work — which is the real key to fitness.

Let me explain. Total work is a combination of how hard, how long, and how often a person exercises. Training requires a *minimum* heart rate threshold (somewhere between 40 and 50 percent of maximum), a minimum number of minutes (about 15 to 20), and a minimum number of days per week (two to four). These factors can be adjusted so that if a person works harder (more intensely), he or she does not need to exercise as long. If a person works at less intensity, he or she needs to exercise longer.

How hard? The best way to determine how hard you should exercise is to measure the maximum amount of oxygen your body is capable of using. To do this, you can ride a specialized bicycle or walk or run on a treadmill (stress test). While you give an all-out effort, a doctor measures the amount of oxygen you use. Since it is a maximum effort, it is called maximum oxygen uptake (max VO2). With this information, the physician can prescribe how hard to exercise. In school your children may be asked to run a mile or so as a fitness test. That test can give the teacher an estimate of your child's maximum oxygen uptake.

If you don't want to go through a stress test, you can use your heart rate as a worthy alternative. Simply reach for your wrist and count your heart rate. (See box.) Then make sure you exercise at a level that keeps your heart beating at the proper rate, which will differ for different people.

Everyone has a maximum heart rate (see

How to Figure Your Heart Rate

The number of times your heart pumps blood each minute is your pulse rate or heart rate. To feel your pulse, sit quietly for three to five minutes. Then turn the palm of your hand up and place two or three fingers of your right hand on the thumb side of your left wrist.

When taking your pulse, you should feel a push or thump against your fingers. Each push is one heart beat, which is called your pulse. The number of pushes each minute is your heart or pulse rate.

After locating your pulse, look at the sweep second hand on your watch. Starting with zero, count the number of beats for a 10-second interval. Multiply that number by 6. This represents your resting heart rate per minute. A normal heart rate for adults after sitting quietly one to five minutes is 54 to 82 beats per minute. With children, heart rates are usually between 72 and 100 beats per minute. Children under ten often will have resting heart rates of 86 to 100.

Table 3). Your maximum heart rate is the number of beats per minute when you are exercising as hard, as fast, and as long as possible. Although it varies from person to person, your maximum heart rate is roughly 220 minus your

TABLE 3
MAXIMUM HEART RATE

Age	Maximum Heart Rate (bpm)*	Age	Maximum Heart Rate (bpm)*
10 or less	210	45	175
15	205	50	170
20	200	55	165
25	195	60	160
30	190	65	155
35	185	70 or more	150
40	180		

*bpm = beats per minute

age. If you are twenty years old, your maximum heart rate is about 200. If you are forty, it's about 180.

Do not try to exercise at your maximum heart rate level. That is not necessary for general fitness. A safe and more appropriate level is between 40 and 75 percent of your maximum. That is your ideal heart rate range.

To find your ideal heart rate range, check your resting pulse. (See box.) Subtract the number of resting beats per minute from your maximum heart rate (on Table 3). That gives you your heart rate range. Multiply your range by 40 to 75 percent and add that number to your resting heart rate. For example, the calculation for a forty-year-old who has a resting heart rate of 60 will look like the rate shown in the box on page 37.

This person's ideal heart rate range would be 108 to 150 beats per minute.

Check your pulse after you have walked, run,

```
180 Maximum heart rate
-60 Resting heart rate
Equals 120 Heart rate range

120 × 40% = 48
  + resting heart rate (60) = 108
120 × 75% = 90
  + resting heart rate (60) = 150
```

biked, swum, cross-country skied, rowed, or aerobicized for at least ten minutes. Count your pulse beats for ten seconds and multiply the number by six to determine your heart beats per minute while exercising.

If your heart rate is higher than your ideal heart rate range, slow your pace or reduce the resistance if you're riding a bike or rowing. If your heart rate is lower than the range, pick up your pace or increase your resistance during the next exercise session. You should push yourself, but not too hard. You should be breathing deeper than usual, and you probably will perspire. The exercise should be pain-free, however, and you should be able to talk to someone next to you (real or imagined) as you exercise.

With children, you can expect the pulse rates of those over ten years old to vary substantially. It also is normal for children under ten to want to stop and go when exercising. That is, run, walk, skip, throw, and go back to running. Let them. The key is to keep their interest. Give them the freedom to move as they want at their own rhythm, but encourage them to keep moving. Additionally, you will need to check their heart rates for them.

How long? When training your heart and lungs, most experts agree that at least 20 minutes of exercise at 60 to 65 percent of your heart rate range is necessary. Of course, the intensity may be increased or decreased. Maybe 50 percent is more comfortable for you. Therefore, you must exercise longer to adjust for the reduced intensity. Table 4 shows how long to exercise, based on pulse rates.

Two notes of caution: First, for healthy, normal people, the training effect on the heart and lungs usually does not occur below 45 percent of a person's maximum heart rate. Second, 30 minutes can be an eternity for children. When exercising as a family, keep their interest by playing games, such as those recommended after this chapter. Also, any efforts to increase the amount of time exercising should be gradual. And if it is clear that 15 minutes is their current attention span, so be it. Take that and don't force them to exercise for longer periods of time.

How often? Exercise a minimum of three to five times a week. Studies show that this provides a reasonable and optimum frequency of exercise.

Now you have it! Walk, run, bike, swim, aerobicize, row, or cross-country ski about an hour at 50 to 75 percent of your maximum heart rate range. Doing this for 15 to 50 minutes three to five times a week will train your heart and lungs, reduce selected cardi-

TABLE 4

NUMBER OF MINUTES OF RECOMMENDED EXERCISE AT DIFFERENT TRAINING HEART RATES

Percent of Maximum Heart Rate	Number of Minutes to Exercise— Heart/Lung Fitness
50%	45:01–52:30
55%	37:31–45:00
60%	30:01–37:30
65%	25:01–30:00
70%	20:01–25:00
75%	15:00–20:00

ovascular risk factors, and energize your body and mind.

STRENGTHENING MUSCLE FITNESS

To improve your muscle fitness, you need to overload your muscles with specific exercises such as calisthenics (push-ups and sit-ups), weight training (free weights), training with equipment (Universal- or Nautilus-type machines), or isometrics. Select whatever approach you prefer. Maybe Mom will prefer weights, and Dad, calisthenics, or vice versa. It doesn't matter. Either will improve your muscle fitness.

I caution you, however, that children who have not reached puberty should avoid training with weights. Some experts feel that young children's bones, tendons, and ligaments are not fully developed. Therefore, they should wait until they are fourteen or so before they begin weight training. Calisthenic training is OK for children eight and above, but those under eight tend not to like it. They are best encouraged by watching Mom and Dad exercising. If they want to jump in and exercise for five minutes, great! Encourage, but don't force.

PUTTING IT ALL TOGETHER

Doing all the things recommended in this chapter may seem overwhelming. Fortunately, it's not. Cardiovascular endurance, muscle fitness, and flexibility can be incorporated into a 30- to 45-minute workout.

Just remember the following four points about each exercise session.

1. The 5- to 10-minute warm-up should include:
   - 2½ to 5 minutes of walking, easy running or doing your cardiovascular exercise at a slow pace;
   - 2½ to 5 minutes of stretching exercises.
2. Exercise aerobically
   - 15 to 52½ minutes of your aerobic exercise (training heart rate), depending upon your exercise intensity.
3. Muscle fitness
   - 10 to 15 minutes of muscle fitness is sufficient. This is an optional aspect of the workout. If you find your muscle fitness to be good, you can skip this part of the workout.
4. The 5- to 10-minute cool-down should include:

- 1 to 5 minutes of slower walking.
- 4 to 5 minutes of stretching exercises.

The minimum amount of time for workouts is 25 minutes three times a week; the maximum is 1½ hours five times a week. That means you will spend one to 4 percent of your time each week exercising. Most people will exercise 2 to 2½ percent of their time. If properly orchestrated, the exercise can double as family time or one-to-one time with your spouse or one of your children. Some of my best conversations with my wife and children have been on long runs or when lifting weights, riding a bicycle, or cross-country skiing.

Often you will find that the children will want to do only one of the four stages of a workout. Or they may do only a few minutes of each. This is fine, since you are planting the seeds for an active life-style later on.

FAMILY FITNESS ACTIVITIES
- No-Sit Day (Ages 5–16)
Select one day (i.e., Saturday) as a no-sitting day. The object of this contest is to go through the whole day, from 9:00 A.M. to 5:00 P.M., without sitting. This activity is fun, but it is tiring (no sitting means no lying down, kneeling, etc. — only standing, walking, or running). See how many family members make it through the day. Discuss the adventure at the evening meal, while sitting.

- Exercise Monopoly (Ages 8–14)
If you have the popular board game Monopoly,

you can adapt it to reinforce exercise concepts. Change all the properties to exercise facilities or places synonymous with fitness. Half the fun will be thinking up new names for the properties (i.e., Fred's Fantastic Fitness Facility, Boston Marathon Route).

You may wish to change the cards as well, to require participants to be active (i.e., run around the room three times, do five push-ups). Every time a person passes "Go" to collect $200 he must do ten sit-ups.

The object of the game is to gain control of all the fitness facilities!

● Family Fitness Cheer (Ages 7–14)
Have a "Family Fitness Cheer" contest to see who can come up with a funny and creative family cheer. You might use the cheer to help motivate family members to get out of bed in the morning.

Sample cheer:

Hey Kuntzlemans
We like the gyms.
Run, jump, and roll;
Fitness is our goal.
Feelin' good, feelin' spry,
That's the way to really try.

● Measuring Your Family's Fitness
   (Ages 6 and Up)
Flexibility: Sit and Reach
Put a piece of tape on the floor. Sit perpendicular to it, with your legs extended and heels

SIT AND REACH TEST NORMS (INCHES)

Age	Sex	Excellent	Average	Improvement Needed
6–9	F	23+	17–22	0–16
	M	22+	13–22	0–12
10–13	F	23+	17–22	0–16
	M	22+	13–21	0–12
14–29	F	23+	17–22	0–16
	M	22+	13–21	0–12
30–39	F	23+	17–22	0–16
	M	22+	13–21	0–12
40–49	F	22+	15–21	0–14
	M	21+	13–20	0–12
50–59	F	21+	14–20	0–13
	M	20+	12–19	0–11
60 and over	F	21+	14–20	0–11
	M	20+	12–19	0–11

about five inches apart, just touching the inside edge of the tape. Place a yardstick between your legs, with the fifteen-inch mark on the inside edge of the tape. As your partner holds your knees straight, reach forward with both hands as far as possible (don't lunge) and touch the stick.

Muscle Fitness: Push-Ups

Women: Keep your shoulders, back and buttocks straight and your knees bent. Place your hands directly under your shoulders. Bend your elbows until your chest touches the floor. Without pausing, do as many as you can.

Men: Ditto, but with straight legs. Lower yourself till your chest touches a friend's upright fist on the floor.

PUSH-UPS TEST NORMS (NUMBER COMPLETED)

Age	Sex	Excellent	Average	Improvement Needed
6–9	F	16 +	9–15	0–8
	M	16 +	16–30	0–8
10–13	F	31 +	0–8	0–15
	M	31 +	0–15	0–15
14–29	F	46 +	17–45	0–16
	M	51 +	25–50	0–24
30–39	F	41 +	12–40	0–11
	M	46 +	22–45	0–21
40–49	F	36 +	8–35	0–7
	M	41 +	19–40	0–18
50–59	F	31 +	6–30	0–5
	M	36 +	15–35	0–14
60 and over	F	26 +	5–25	0–4
	M	31 +	10–30	0–9

Curl-Ups

Lie flat with your knees bent and heels six inches from your buttocks. Place your hands on your thighs. While a partner holds down your feet, curl up your head, then shoulders, then upper trunk. Come up until your fingertips touch the middle of your kneecaps, then return. Do as many as you can without pausing.

CURL-UPS TEST NORMS (NUMBER COMPLETED)

Age	Sex	Excellent	Average	Improvement Needed
6–9	F	15 +	10–14	0–5
	M	15 +	10–14	0–5
10–13	F	41 +	21–40	0–20
	M	41 +	21–40	0–20
14–29	F	46 +	25–45	0–24
	M	51 +	30–50	0–29
30–39	F	41 +	20–40	0–19
	M	46 +	22–45	0–21

Age	Sex	Excellent	Average	Improvement Needed
40–49	F	36 +	16–35	0–15
	M	41 +	21–40	0–20
50–59	F	31 +	12–30	0–11
	M	36 +	18–35	0–17
60 and over	F	26 +	11–25	0–10
	M	31 +	15–30	0–14

Cardiovascular Fitness: Step Test

Facing a twelve-inch high bench, step one foot on top, then the other, then down with one foot and then the other. Pace is critical—do twenty-four full steps a minute. Go for 3 minutes, then sit down immediately. Have your partner count your heart rate for one minute starting 5 seconds after you finish the exercise.

3-MINUTE STEP TEST NORMS (HEART RATE)

Age	Sex	Excellent	Average	Improvement Needed
6–9	F	100 or less	100–119	120 +
	M	100 or less	100–119	120 +
10–13	F	92 or less	93–113	114 +
	M	92 or less	93–113	114 +
14–29	F	to 79	80–110	111 +
	M	to 74	75–100	101 +
30–39	F	to 83	84–115	116 +
	M	to 77	78–109	110 +
40–49	F	to 87	88–118	119 +
	M	to 79	80–112	113 +
50–59	F	to 91	92–123	124 +
	M	to 89	85–115	116 +
60 and over	F	to 94	95–127	128 +
	M	to 89	90–118	119 +

CHAPTER
3

Eating Well to Live Right

Today *nutrition* has become a kind of gospel word. Good nutrition is a lifesaver, a blessing to good health. But too often, confusing messages about food and drink bombard us. They look good; they sound right; they are very appealing; but alas, they may be bad news indeed. We need knowledge and discernment. This chapter can help.

NUTRIENTS—ESSENTIAL TO LIFE

Nutritionists tell us there are six basic nutrients: carbohydrates, fats, proteins, vitamins, minerals, and water. All six nutrients are essential for your family's health, vitality, and appearance.

Foods are composed of these nutrients. For example, a piece of beef includes proteins, fats, small amounts of carbohydrates, vitamins, minerals, and water. Carrots contain carbohydrates, vitamins, minerals, water, and a trace of proteins. Table sugar is almost 100 percent carbohydrates.

Let's look more closely at the six nutrients.

Health Hazard: Cancer

One out of every four Americans will develop some kind of cancer. Barring new breakthroughs in cancer research, about 60 percent of these people will die of this disease.

Essentially, cancer is a degenerative disease of the cells. The DNA (material coded with information as to what the cell can do and its offspring can become) changes, causing the growth regulation of the affected cells to go haywire. These cells divide abnormally. The cancerous cells, as they are called, injure the body by crowding out normal cells and robbing them of their nutrients. The abnormal cells tend to form masses called tumors.

As in the case of heart disease, the key to battling cancer seems to be in prevention. Researchers say that 60 percent of all cancers could be prevented if people:[1]

- stopped smoking
- avoided overexposure to sunlight
- dropped their weight and body fat
- ate foods rich in fiber and vitamins C, A, and E
- ate less sugar and fat
- avoided alcohol and drugs
- reduced their stress
- avoided unnecessary X rays and exposure to noxious gases, nitrates and nitrites (found in hotdogs, bacon, and luncheon meats), and selected chemicals (plastics, coal tar, dyes, arsenic, and pesticides)

TABLE 5
COMPLEX CARBOHYDRATES AND "HEALTHFUL" SIMPLE CARBOHYDRATES

Fructose (Healthful Simple Carbohydrates)

Apples	Grapes	Pears
Apricots	Guava	Persimmons
Bananas	Kumquats	Pineapple
Blackberries	Lemon juice	Plums
Blueberries	Loganberries	Pomegranates
Breadfruit	Lychees	Quinces
Cherries	Mangoes	Raisins
Cranberries	Muskmelons	Raspberries
Dates	Nectarines	Strawberries
Figs	Oranges	Tangerines
Gooseberries	Papayas	Watermelon
Grapefruit	Peaches	

Complex Carbohydrates
Grains

Barley	Oatmeal	Rye
Buckwheat	Popcorn	Wheat
Cornmeal	Rice	

Vegetables

Artichokes	Corn kernels	Peas
Asparagus	Cucumbers	Peppers
Bamboo	Eggplant	Potatoes
shoots	Endive	Pumpkins
Bean sprouts	Garbanzos	Radishes
Beans, snap	Garlic	Rutabagas
green and	Leeks	Squash
yellow	Legumes	Sweet
Beans, lima	(dried)	potatoes
Beans, pinto	Lentils	Swiss chard
Beets	Lettuce	Tapioca
Broccoli	Mustard	Tomatoes
Cabbage, raw	greens	Turnips
Carrots, raw	Okra	Water
Cauliflower	Onions	chestnuts
Celery	Parsley	
Chives	Parsnips	

Carbohydrates. Carbohydrates are your body's most preferred nutrient. Aside from providing energy, high-quality carbohydrate foods contain important minerals and vitamins.

Carbohydrates come in the form of sugars, starches, or cellulose. Sugars sometimes are called simple carbohydrates, which include fruits, food made with sugar (cakes, jam, cookies), table sugar, and honey. Starches are called complex carbohydrates (see Table 5). Cellulose, often called fiber, is a complex carbohydrate that is difficult to digest. It is important in keeping the digestive tract healthy. High cellulose foods include bran, whole grains, and vegetables and fruits with seeds and skin.

Fats. Fats are a class of nutrients made up of fatty acids and glycerin (an organic alcohol). They are found in foods such as butter and other dairy products, meats, salad and cooking oils, chocolate, and peanut butter. Pound for pound, fats provide more usable energy than carbohydrates or proteins. They also take longer to digest, so you feel fuller after a meal or a snack that contains some kind of fatty component.

The fatty acids that constitute fats are of three general kinds: saturated, unsaturated, and polyunsaturated. The less hydrogen present, the more unsaturated the fat is.

Proteins. Your body uses proteins to build and repair body tissues. If your protein supply is not sufficient to offset the daily destruction of cells, your body begins to waste away. A poor protein diet has serious effects on growth and development.

TABLE 6

THREE TYPES OF FAT

Saturated
beef
butter
cheese (whole milk)
chocolate
coconut
cream
ice cream
lamb
margarine (regular)
milk (whole)
pork
shortening (hydrogenated)
veal

Unsaturated	*Polyunsaturated*
almonds	corn oil
cashews	fish
chicken (not skin)	herring oil
olive oil	special margarine
peanuts	safflower oil
peanut oil	soybean oil
pecans	walnuts
turkey	wheat germ oil

Proteins are present in all living tissues. Protein molecules are composed of many nitrogen-containing components called amino acids. There are twenty-one amino acids, of which your body can manufacture eleven. The other ten, called essential amino acids, can be obtained only by eating the right foods.

Proteins are crucial, but they are not required in large amounts. Meat, fish, and eggs are rich in complete protein. They contain all

TABLE 7

PROTEIN FOODS

Animal Products (Complete Protein)

Beef	Duck	Milk
Cheese	Eggs	Pork
Chicken	Fish	Turkey

Grains (Incomplete Protein)

Brown rice	Oats
Corn	Rice

Legumes (Incomplete Protein)

Garbanzo beans	Peas
Kidney beans	Soy sprouts
Lima beans	Soybean flour
Mung beans	Soybeans

Nuts and Seeds (Incomplete Protein)

Cashews
Peanuts

Vegetarian Dishes* (Complete Protein Dishes)

Barley and yogurt soup
Bean or pea curry on rice
Blended dip of garbanzos, sesame, lemon, garlic, oil
Bread made with milk or cheese
Breads with added seed meals
Breads with sesame or sunflower seed spread
Cereal with milk
Cheese sandwiches
Cheese sauce, garbanzo beans
Corn-soy bread

*Each of these dishes combines nonmeat protein foods (those not containing all ten essential amino acids) to make a complete protein dish—one that provides all the essential amino acids.

Corn tortillas and beans
Legume soup with bread
Lentil curry on rice
Macaroni and cheese
Middle Eastern hummus (sesame and
  chick-peas)
Milk in legume soups
Pasta with milk or cheese
Pea soup and toast
Rice and milk pudding
Rice-bean casserole
Rice-cheese casserole
Rice with sesame seeds
Sesame salt on legume dish
Sesame seeds in bean soups and casseroles
Sunflower seeds and peanuts
Wheat berries with cheese sauce
Wheat bread with baked beans
Wheat-soy bread

Source: Based on Frances Lappe, *Diet for a Small Planet*
(New York: Ballantine, 1975).

the essential amino acids. Cereals, breads,
nuts, and most fruits and vegetables contain
lesser amounts and incomplete proteins, which
means that they do not contain all ten essential amino acids. For most effective use by our
bodies, they should be combined with other
proteins (see Table 7).

Vitamins. Vitamins make it possible for you
to use appropriately the food you eat. They
provide for chemical control of body functions
and play an important role in energy production, normal growth, resistance to infection,
and general health.

The highest sources of vitamins are meats,
particularly the liver and kidneys; fruits; vege-

The Vitamin Controversy

There is much controversy regarding the amount of vitamins needed by Americans. On one side of the coin, the traditional medical establishment advocates the United States government recommended daily allowances (RDA) on vitamins. On the other side of the coin, some famous biochemists, such as Drs. Linus Pauling and Roger Williams, recommend megavitamins. Megavitamins are large doses of certain vitamins to reduce the incidence of disease—everything from the common cold to cancer.

Quite frankly, the vitamin story is far from complete. Research findings have not been definitive. Most of the studies show that supplementing an already well-balanced diet will not improve health. But, and it's a big one, most of these studies have been conducted over relatively short periods of time. We don't know what effect vitamin supplementation has (good or bad) over a ten-, fifteen-, or twenty-year period of time.

Research *has* demonstrated that certain people need extra vitamins. Heavy alcohol drinkers, heavy smokers, and women who are using a birth control pill seem to have difficulty securing enough vitamins from food. You cannot assume, however, that if a little of a vitamin is good for you, a lot is better. When your cells are vitamin-saturated, additional vitamins are worthless.

tables; milk; eggs; fish; and certain cereals. Vitamin deficiencies can result in night blindness, poor bone and tooth formation, scurvy, stunted growth, lack of vitality, poor condition of skin and mucous membranes, and a loss of appetite and weight.

Minerals. Minerals are inorganic chemical substances. Like vitamins, they are important in regulating body functions and are essential to the structure of bones and other body tissues.

For years, nutritionists have emphasized the major minerals—calcium, magnesium, phosphorus, potassium, sodium, and sulfur. More recently, work begun by Dr. Henry A. Schroeder, professor emeritus at Dartmouth Medical School, has demonstrated that trace minerals, although present in minute amounts, are essential for normal metabolism. Trace minerals include chromium, copper, fluorine, iodine, iron, manganese, selenium, and zinc.

Water. Water accounts for about 70 percent of the body's weight. It is acquired in three ways: taken as drink, contained in foods we eat, and formed within the body as a result of the oxidation process. Water is lost from the body through urination, defecation, perspiration, and evaporation. In the average adult, daily water loss amounts to about three quarts, so we must replace that amount daily. Two quarts of that requirement are provided by the food we eat. We must drink the rest.

THE BASIC FOUR—OR SEVEN?

Nutritionists have reduced all of this information into a palatable approach for the average family by creating the four basic food groups:

Group 1: The vegetable-fruit group
Group 2: The bread-cereal group
Group 3: The milk group
Group 4: The meat group

To insure adequate intake of the six nutrients, they recommend eating daily:

- Four servings of group 1 (vegetables-fruits)
- Four servings of group 2 (breads-cereals)
- Two or three servings of group 3 (milk)
- Two servings of group 4 (meat)

Alas, this plan is unsatisfactory. According to Jean Mayer, Ph.D., world-famous nutritionist and currently president of Tufts University, "There is no reason, for example, to classify potatoes and spinach together. It would make more sense to gather the main sources of animal protein and good quality vegetable proteins (milk, meat, fish, eggs, peas, and beans) and separate starch fruits (bananas) and roots (potatoes) from green leafy vegetables and other foods."[2]

Because of Dr. Mayer's criteria and my own work with helping people eat a more healthy diet, I propose the following food classification system:

Group 1: Non-starchy vegetables (basically, green or leafy vegetables)

TABLE 8 — NUTRITION GUIDE

Group	Score	Food Groups & Number of Servings	Day 1	Day 2	Day 3
1	20	Two servings (about 1 cup) of non-starch vegetables (basically leafy/green, such as asparagus and zucchini).			
2	10	One serving (about ½ cup) or starch vegetables, such as corn and potatoes.			
3	10	One serving (about ½ cup) of fruit—citrus or non-citrus.			
4	20	Two cups of milk or milk products. One-inch cube of cheese is equivalent to ½ cup of milk.			
5	20	Two servings (total: approximately 4 oz.) of protein food (meat, poultry, fish, dried beans, peas, nuts, eggs, or vegetable dishes listed on Table 7).			
6	20	Four or more servings of grain products (breads, cereals, or noodles).			
7	0	Zero servings of fats, sweets, and alcohol.			

Group 2: Starchy vegetables (basically, white and yellow vegetables)

Group 3: Fruits

Group 4: Milk and milk products

Group 5: Protein foods

Group 6: Grain foods

Group 7: Fats, sweets, and alcohol

To insure adequate intake of the six nutrients, you should eat daily:

- Two servings from Group 1
- One serving from Group 2
- One serving from Group 3
- Two servings from Group 4
- Two servings from Group 5
- Four servings from Group 6
- Zero servings from Group 7

This approach allows you to obtain a wide source of vitamins and minerals. It also requires you to diversify your eating plan.

While this guide gives you an indication of whether or not you are getting a sufficient amount of nutrients, it does not take into account the saturated fat, sugar, fiber, and salt in your diet. We'll discuss those shortly.

HOW WELL DOES YOUR FAMILY EAT?

Many people think their family eats well. The "Nutrition Guide" (Table 8) gives you important guidelines for determining your family's and your own eating habits.

The guide is simple to use. If you eat what is recommended for each group, you receive the maximum number of points. For example, if you eat two servings of non-starchy vegetables, you receive 20 points. If you eat one serving, you get 10 points. If you don't eat any, you get zero. Follow this pattern for all the groups.

After you finish, total your score. If you get 100 points (the maximum score), you will be getting the recommended daily allowance for vitamins, minerals, fats, proteins, and carbohydrates. If you fall below 100, you are deficient in one or more of these categories.

Take the test now, then have your spouse and children do likewise. If the children are too young or you anticipate resistance, do it for them. Watch their eating for a day (don't tell them what you're doing). You may be surprised!

SIX FOODS TO AVOID

Sugar. The average American adult eats 2 to slightly less than 2½ pounds of sugar a week, which breaks down to 500 to 600 calories per day of pure sugar. That is too much. It amounts to 18 percent of a person's total calorie consumption. Our studies on children in grades two through seven showed that the average child eats 25 percent of his or her calories from simple carbohydrates, mostly from pop, candy, donuts, "ade" drinks, presweetened cereals, etc.

All of this is particularly serious because a diet high in sucrose usually tends to be low in other basic nutrients—especially the B vitamins and several essential minerals. Additionally, the sugar comes highly refined and stripped of any fiber, which is necessary for a healthy intestinal tract. A diet high in sugar has been linked to heart disease, tooth decay, diabetes, hypoglycemia, fatigue, obesity, cancer, arthritis, and hyperactivity.

While sugar may taste good, moderation is the key. A reasonable intake is 200 to 250 calories a day—about a pound of sugar a week.

Fats. We Americans consume more fat per person than any other nation in the world. In fact, we eat 80 percent of the world's foods that are high in saturated fat.

Fats can be a source of energy, but when eaten to excess, problems occur. According to many scientists, the fats you eat actually can suffocate your tissues by depriving them of oxygen. A diet high in fat also can raise blood cholesterol levels. This cholesterol tends to be deposited on the lining of the arteries, partially blocking them so less oxygen gets to the heart and the likelihood of heart disease increases.

Now the distinction between saturated, unsaturated, and polyunsaturated fats (see Table 6) becomes important. Excessive intake of saturated fat tends to raise the level of cholesterol in the blood. Unsaturated fats are considered "neutral fats," since they neither raise nor lower the level of cholesterol in the blood. But polyunsaturated oils tend to lower cholesterol levels.

Cholesterol. Cholesterol is a fat-like substance present in all animal tissues, such as blood, muscle, liver, and brain. It is both manufactured by the body and found in all foods of animal origin. Eggs, organ meats, and

TABLE 9

CHOLESTEROL CONTENT OF COMMON FOODS

Foods	Amount (Cooked)	Cholesterol (mg)
Brains	3 oz.	2000
Kidney, all kinds	3 oz.	683
Liver, chicken	3 oz.	634
Liver, beef	3 oz.	372
Egg yolk	1	272
Heart, beef	3 oz.	233
Shrimp	3 oz.	128
Cream cheese	3 oz.	94
Cheddar cheese	3 oz.	90
Veal	3 oz.	86
Crab	3 oz.	85
Beef, lean	3 oz.	77
Chicken drumstick, without skin	3 oz.	77
Pork, lean	3 oz.	75
American cheese	3 oz.	75
Lobster	3 oz.	72
Chicken breast, without skin	3 oz.	67
Clams, canned	3 oz.	54
Flounder	3 oz.	50
Oysters	3 oz.	50
Milk, whole	1 cup	34
Milk, low-fat (2%)	1 cup	18
Milk, low-fat (1%)	1 cup	10
Milk, nonfat (skim)	1 cup	5
Fruits, vegetables, and grains	Any amount	0

Source: Jane Brody, *Jane Brody's Nutrition Book* (New York: W. W. Norton, 1981), 83-84.

shrimp contain more cholesterol than any other animal products.

Keeping blood cholesterol levels low is important for you and your children. Dr. Gerald

Berenson of Louisiana State University Medical College in New Orleans has traced children's blood cholesterol levels over the past fourteen years. Not surprisingly, about one-half of the people who had high blood cholesterol levels as children have elevated blood cholesterol levels later in life.[3]

Salt. Before we discuss salt, we need to distinguish between sodium and sodium chloride. Sodium is a trace mineral found naturally in many foods. Your body needs regular, small amounts of sodium. Sodium chloride is a chemically manufactured salt, commonly referred to as table salt.

The average person probably needs no more than a gram of salt a day, yet many Americans eat between eight and fifteen grams of table salt daily. We plaster it on pretzels, popcorn, peanuts, potato chips, and French fries.

Table salt may cause hypertension or high blood pressure if you are salt- or sodium-sensitive. Again, Dr. Berenson's study provides important information. Children who eat a lot of salty foods are more likely to have high blood pressure now and when they are older.[4]

Caffeine. Every morning, about 80 percent of America's adult population chugs a mug or two of coffee. By noon a good share of those 100 million people have had two to five cups.

Experiments indicate that the caffeine in coffee increases mental alertness, speeds reaction time, and helps people think more clearly. In short, caffeine buzzes the brain and nervous system, perhaps by increasing the concentration of a hormone stimulator called cyclic AMP, which increases alertness.

Most coffee drinkers want this effect, but they realize they don't get it from a cup or two of coffee. One cup of coffee generally contains only 100 to 150 milligrams of caffeine, a relatively harmless amount. The average coffee drinker goes through two to three cups a day, however, pushing the amount of caffeine to 200 to 450 milligrams. They also may get caffeine from other sources, such as tea, cola drinks, or cocoa. Compounding the problem, their bodies develop an immunity to those boosts in alertness and reaction time. That is why the two- to three-cups-a-day coffee drinkers easily can increase their consumption to six to eight cups, which provides close to 1000-milligrams of caffeine. That level can produce dizziness, restlessness, irritability, and tremors.

Children are not immune to caffeine. Your children may not drink coffee, but they may drink colas, iced tea, cocoa, and chocolate milk. They also probably eat chocolate candy. Two cola drinks and a glass of chocolate milk contain 130 to 170 milligrams of caffeine. For a seven-year-old, that is equivalent to drinking four to six cups of brewed coffee.

Excessive caffeine consumption has been associated with heart and kidney diseases, skipped heart beats, cancer, gastric upsets, anxiety, and insomnia.

Additives. Additives preserve the freshness of food and enhance its flavor and color. Currently, more than 5,000 different kinds of additives are used to process the food we eat.

Practically every food you eat contains some type of additive. That doesn't mean practically everything you eat is bad. Some additives are necessary and do not adversely affect your health. Other additives may present health hazards.

Avoid (or be cautious about) foods that contain the following additives: artificial colorings blue No. 1, blue No. 2, citrus red No. 2, green No. 3, red No. 40, and yellow No. 5; brominated vegetable oil (BVO); caffeine (for children and pregnant women); monosodium glutamate (MSG) (for children and adults); quinine; saccharin; sodium nitrate; and sodium nitrite. These additives have been poorly tested and serve no essential role. Some studies have been demonstrated that there may be some risk in using products containing them.

You also should be cautious about the following as they, too, have been inadequately researched and safer substitutes are available: artificial coloring yellow No. 6; artificial flavorings; butylated hydroxyanisole (BHA); butylated hydroxytoluene (BHT); caffeine (for nonpregnant adults); carrageenan; heptylparaben; mono and diglycerides; phosphoric acid and phosphates; propyl gallate; sodium bisulfite; and sulfur dioxide.

THE BASIC SEVEN QUESTIONS
The discussion of sugar, salt, fat, cholesterol, caffeine, and additives brings us back to the seven basic food groups. The basic seven leave a lot of unanswered questions. Here are a few:

Healthy Eating Pays Off

A slight shift in eating habits to less cholesterol, fat, sugar, salt, and calories would result in:[5]

- 1.2 million fewer cases of heart and vascular disease each year
- 64,000 fewer cancer deaths and 120,000 fewer cases of cancer each year
- 49 million fewer cases of respiratory infection
- 3 million fewer cases of birth defects
- 3 million fewer cases of arthritis
- 3 million fewer cases of osteoporosis (thinning of the bones)
- 16,200 fewer cases of blindness
- 3 million fewer cases of allergies
- 2.5 million fewer mental health problems requiring hospitalization

1. May I eat canned or frozen fruits and vegetables?

2. May I count ice cream as one of the servings of milk? What about whole milk or cream?

3. What kinds of meats should I serve? Are luncheon meats, hotdogs, or hamburgers OK?

4. Do foods such as white breads, cakes, pies, granola bars, and cookies qualify as grain products?

5. How do I cut our fat, cholesterol, sugar, caffeine, and salt intake?

6. Are we to eat from the first six food groups before we are permitted to eat from the

seventh, which contains soda pop, coffee, candy, and alcohol?

7. What about combination foods, such as pizza, macaroni and cheese, TV dinners, meatless bacon, egg substitutes, and so on?

These are important questions. Let me try to answer them.

1. Avoid canned fruits and vegetables. Canning may cause a loss of vitamins. Peas, for example, may lose 38 percent of their vitamins in the canning process. Plus, most cans of vegetables have one-half to one gram of sodium or salt added.

2. Ice cream and ice milk are high in fat and cholesterol. They are also rich in sugar. Therefore, I do not permit ice cream or ice milk as part of the milk group. They belong in group 7. Whole milk is also not to be included. Only low-fat (2 percent or less) milk products qualify.

3. Lean meats, poultry, and fish are acceptable. Luncheon meats are a no-no.

4. Cakes, pies, granola bars, cookies, and crackers are unusually high in sugar, fat, possible cholesterol, and salt. White bread is permitted only in a pinch. Whole grain products are recommended.

5. The recommendations made in items 1 to 4 above will allow you to meet the U.S. recommendations on fat, salt, cholesterol, sugar, and fiber.

6. Soda pop, coffee, and candy are permitted on occasion (a total of one to three times a week).

7. Combination foods, such as pizza, macaroni and cheese, and so on, must be viewed with caution. While they may provide you with vitamins, minerals, protein, and other nutrients, they also tend to give you heavy doses of salt, saturated fat, cholesterol, and sugar. Furthermore, it has been reported that from the time a frozen TV dinner is prepared at the company until you take it out of your oven and place it on your table, 40 percent of its vitamin A, 100 percent of its vitamin C, 80 percent of its B12-complex vitamins, and 55 percent of its vitamin E have been lost.

THE BASIC SEVEN – MODIFIED

Because of all the problems associated with salt, sugar, fat, cholesterol, caffeine, and additives, I suggest that my seven basic food groups be modified as follows:

Group 1: Two servings (approximately 1 cup) of fresh or frozen green or leafy vegetables (non-starchy). No canned vegetables.

Group 2: One serving (½ cup) of fresh or frozen white or yellow vegetable (starchy). *No canned vegetables*.

Group 3: One serving (½ cup) of fresh or frozen (no sugar added) fruit. No canned fruit.

Group 4: Two servings (2 cups total) of low-fat milk or milk products. Lowfat is 2 percent or less.

Group 5: Two servings of protein foods. These

include lean red meat, poultry, fish, beans, lentils, and eggs (no yolks). Fish and poultry are not to be breaded.

Group 6: Four servings of whole grain breads, cereals (no added sugars), or grains.

Group 7: One serving of sugar or fat (unsaturated or polyunsaturated oil) per meal.

Now that you know how to modify the basic seven foods, go back to Table 8. Take the test again without counting canned or high-fat foods or white bread. How do you and your family fare? If your score is the same as before, congratulations (provided, of course, that you received 100 points). If the modified score is lower (it probably will be), examine the table closely and see where you can make improvements.

FOOD PURCHASING STRATEGIES

1. Buy salt-free potato chips (taste good) and pretzels (taste fair to good).

2. Salt-free soups and vegetables are available. Most popular brands are pretty weak, but you can season them to your taste.

3. Buy canned fruit packed in its own juice.

4. Purchase fruit juices, rather than fruit drinks. Check labels. Preferred—no sugar added, rather than unsweetened or sweetened.

5. Purchase canned fish (i.e., tuna) packed in water, rather than oil.

6. Never eat presweetened cereals. The following cereals have 10 percent or less sugar:

Grape Nuts
Shredded Wheat (large biscuit)
Shredded Wheat (spoon size)
Wheat Germ
Cheerios
Puffed Rice
Uncle Sam Cereal
Wheat Chex
Cream of Rice (hot)
Farina (hot)
Old-Fashioned Quaker Oats (hot)
Instant Quaker Oatmeal (hot)
Grape Nut Flakes
Puffed Wheat
Alpen
Wheatina (hot)
Post Toasties
Product 19
Corn Total
Special K
Wheaties
Cream of Wheat (hot)
Instant Cream of Wheat (hot)
Corn Flakes (Kroger)
Peanut Butter
Corn Flakes (Food Club)
Crispy Rice
Corn Chex
Corn Flakes (Kellogg)
Total
Rice Chex
Crisp Rice
Raisin Bran (Skinner)
Concentrate

7. Select vegetable oils that are not hardened, hydrogenated, or partly hardened or hydrogenated.

8. Select soft tub margarines over hard margarine, or butter.

9. Select low-fat (2 to ½ percent) or skim milk and cheese products.

10. Remember: If it comes in a bag, box, or jar, beware. Read all labels carefully.

11. Buy whole-grain flour to use in baking. (Be cautious: "whole wheat" may mean nothing more than wheat-refined.)

12. Buy a whole-grain cereal or whole-grain bread. Try whole-grain pastas and crackers.

13. Regularly buy fruit for snacks and desserts. Reduce the amount of sweetened soft drinks and candy you buy.

14. Purchase more fish and poultry, less red meat.

15. Limit rich desserts to special occasions.

FAMILY FOOD ACTIVITIES
● Snacks (Ages 10–14)

On one sheet of paper, write the heading "Junk Food Hall of Shame" and on another, "Health Food Hall of Fame." Now go through your refrigerator and cupboards and list on these sheets all the foods you have available for snacking. After you finish, post the Health Food Hall of Fame list in a conspicuous place in the kitchen as an advertisement for nutritious snacks. You can add to this list from week to week. Also post the Hall of Shame list.

When family members go a whole week without eating a specific Hall of Shame item, they can put their initial by that item. At the end of a month, see who has initialed the most Hall of Shame items. (This means they have eaten the least amount of junk food.) Have children initial the Health Food Hall of Fame foods they have eaten.

● Nutritious Foods (Ages 3–16)

Have each family member select two nutritious foods (one must be a vegetable) they like. Each week, incorporate these favorite nutritious foods into the weekly menu (e.g., Tuesday is Johnny's day, so we're having cauliflower and yogurt). The following week, family members select two different items. This allows everyone to have input into the weekly menu. It also gets them to try different foods.

● TV Advertising (Ages 8–16)

Discuss with your children the advertising techniques used to sell food, soda pop, cereals, candy, and so on. Does the ad tell the entire truth? The ad may say the soda pop has no caffeine, but you are not told that it is high in sugar and sodium and has no nutritional value.

View the ad, then read the ingredients on the label. Talk about hidden messages and facts. Discussing some of the absurdities implied in television ads can make great dinner conversation.

● Family Garden (Ages 6–16)

Plant a family garden—good exercise and nutrition and fun. Here are some handy suggestions:[6]

1. Plant just enough for your family — avoid being overwhelmed the first year. Later, you can expand.
2. Plant crops that are easy to tend, taste good, and are hard to get — or expensive in stores. Some ideas:
   - leaf lettuce
   - spinach
   - sugar snap peas
   - tomatoes
   - cucumbers
   - herbs (to use fresh)
   - Alpine strawberries
   - blueberries
   - raspberries

Watching Your Weight

Remember the last time you backpacked, climbed a mountain, or carried a suitcase through an airport terminal? After a short time, you wanted to rest. The first thing you did when you stopped was take the pack off your back or put down the suitcase. Why? Your muscles ached. They were screaming for rest and more oxygen.

Now imagine carrying a twenty- to thirty-pound backpack each day. Your different body systems — muscular, skeletal, circulatory, and hormonal — would be under a greater strain to support the additional load. Your body would soon rebel.

It's no different with fat. Excess fat is considered a "pack on the back." Your bones and muscles strain to support the additional load. Your heart and lungs work harder to assist your muscles in moving all the fat around. Scientists tell us that a person who carries too much fat generally takes two to three more breaths per minute, even when sleeping. This is 2,800 to 4,400 more breaths per day.

Health Hazard: Obesity

Government reports show that each decade we are getting fatter. Consider these facts:

- Americans gain an average of one to two pounds a year from age twenty to age fifty.
- 20% of the children six to nine years of age have excess body fat.
- More than 10 million children up to age eighteen carry too much fat.
- More than $50 million is spent each year on diet and exercise books.
- More than $6 million is spent on diet drinks.
- More than $200 million is spent on diet pills.

Obesity seems to stay with people. An obese child usually becomes an obese teenager and adult. Dr. William Clarke, a researcher from the University of Iowa, investigated cardiovascular disease risk factors among children in Muscatine, Iowa. He said, "Well over half of our kids who were overweight in the first grade are overweight when they reach high school."[1]

But obesity can be prevented by:

- Exercising vigorously at least four times a week
- Changing eating habits gradually, as well as moderately reducing calories (200 per day)
- Consuming less alcohol
- Dealing positively with stress
- Minimizing television watching

The extra fat problem goes beyond extra breaths and heart beats and tired muscles and bones. A committee convened by the National Institutes of Health says anyone 20 percent overweight, as determined by life insurance height/weight tables, needs medical help because obesity is a disease. Dr. Jules Hirsch, the committee chairman says, "It is a disease, and it carries with it the risk for increased mortality."[2]

Obesity, according to the committee, is clearly associated with high blood pressure, abnormally high levels of cholesterol in the blood, adult diabetes, and increased risk of cancers of the colon, rectum, and prostate in men, and cancers of the gall bladder, bile passages, breast, cervix, uterus, and ovaries in women.

Fatness goes beyond these physical problems. It causes emotional problems. Self-concepts and relationships have been destroyed by unwanted bulges and bumps.

WEIGHT MANAGEMENT:
A SIMPLE MODEL

The word *calorie* represents a unit of energy. The unit can be used to express either the amount of energy stored in food (one apple has 75 calories) or the amount of energy required to sustain life's activities (sleeping uses one calorie per minute, walking uses 5 calories per minute, for example).

Energy stored in food is consumed as "fuel,"

and in order to provide the energy required to sustain life, your body tries to keep a fine balance between the number of calories you eat and the number of calories you "burn" through daily activities. For example, if you eat 2,000 calories in food each day and use 2,000 calories through activity, you are in a caloric balance and your weight will remain constant.

On the other hand, if you eat 2,000 calories and burn only 1,900, you are in trouble. You have an extra 100 calories. What happens to the 100 calories? The liver converts them into fat. The blood then carries this fat to the various fat cells of your body, where it is stored. While 100 calories doesn't sound like much, if you follow this pattern for thirty-five days, it will amount to 3,500 calories, which is one pound of fat. If you gain one pound of fat every thirty-five days, you will gain approximately ten pounds by the end of one year!

Weight management, then, is simply understanding three important points: (1) Your weight remains the same when you balance calories expended through sleep, work, and play with the calories you eat. (2) Your weight increases when the calories you expend are less than the calories you eat. (3) Your weight decreases when the calories you expend are greater than the calories you eat.

FIVE REASONS DIETS DON'T WORK

If you wish to lose fat and weight, you have three choices: eat less; move more; or eat less

Health Hazards: Anorexia and Bulimia

Two new health concerns have entered the family picture—anorexia nervosa and bulimia. Ninety percent of anorexics and bulimics are women, particularly teenage or young women.

Anorexia nervosa is self-starving. The woman (or, rarely, the man) gradually starts to eat less and exercise more. Her behavior becomes so compulsive that she may exercise two to eight hours a day and eat or drink nothing but diet pop and water. Soon her weight drops—weights of eighty pounds or less are not uncommon.

Anorexia is a big league problem and not to be treated lightly. Most anorexics are perfectionists. For several reasons, they feel that they don't measure up to society's demands for slimness. Consequently, they get caught in a passion to lose weight. They are driven by an obsessive fear of being fat, and they have wildly distorted views of their bodies—picturing themselves as fat, even though they are extremely thin.

Bulimics, on the other hand, gorge on food. They may consume more than 30,000 calories in a day—or even at a sitting—and then purge themselves by inducing vomiting or taking diuretics and laxatives.

Bulimics' eating patterns are bizarre. Some have eaten all the food in the refrigerator at a sitting, eaten the food out of the cat's or dog's dish, or rummaged through garbage cans to find food. Then they move to the bathroom and vomit or excrete all that was eaten. Some bulimics are thin, some are quite heavy, and some yo-yo in weight.

Eating disorders such as anorexia or bulimia stem from a society that equates success with thinness. And they take root as early as seven years of age. We conducted a study regarding self-esteem and body fat and found that many young girls based their self-esteem on slimness.

Not all women were meant to be thin. It is necessary, but difficult, for the bulimic or anorexic to recognize and internalize this truth. They also must learn not to base their self-worth on how they look, nor establish their self-esteem by comparing themselves to someone else—movie stars, models, etc. They must become comfortable with their self-image.

Josh McDowell, in his book *His Image . . . My Image,* explains, "A healthy self-image is seeing yourself as God sees you—no more and no less. . . ."[3]

And how does God view us?

- We are the peak of His creation (Gen. 1:26-27).
- We were created a little lower than the angels (Heb. 2:7).

- God sent His Son to die for us (Mark 10:45).

  We are special. We are loved. If only young people would understand and internalize this. God does not evaluate them on how they look. Neither should they.

and move more. All three will put you into a calorie deficit, so you will lose weight. But not all three are equal.

Dieting is the most common way people try to lose fat. But experts report that only 5 to 10 percent of the obese are able to lose the appropriate fat weight and keep it off through dieting. The great percentage of dieters regain the lost pounds quickly, usually within a few weeks.[4]

Why don't diets work? There are five basic reasons.

1. *Hard work*. Dieting is no fun. Most people don't have the Spartan will that their highly-restrictive diet regimen requires.

2. *Addiction to food*. Some people are emotionally addicted to food. When they are under stress, they eat excessive amounts of food and gain weight. Then they diet, which increases their stress. When the stress becomes acute, they go back on their eating binge, which causes them to be more upset. They are caught in a tragic cycle of stress, eating, depression, guilt, dieting, stress, and more eating.

3. *Social pressure.* Eating is a fundamental aspect of nearly every American social gathering. At parties we enjoy cheese, snacks, nuts, pretzels; at sporting events, hot dogs and soft drinks; at weddings, cake and punch; and at birthdays, cake and ice cream. How can dieters hope to be successful when, at every turn, society strongly reinforces that we are expected to eat—and to eat too much?

4. *The set point theory.* It has been known for several years that dieting decreases the basal metabolic rate (BMR)—the rate at which we burn calories to sustain life. The body also can increase the basal metabolic rate when excessive amounts of food are eaten.

The new set point theory expands upon these two principles in explaining the dieter's plight. According to this theory, the body operates on a type of internal standard, or set point, which dictates the percentage of fat that should be maintained. Obese individuals have high set points and their lean counterparts have low set points.[5]

Regardless of your set point, when your fat content falls below it, your body responds by increasing your appetite. If you do not eat additional food, your BMR decreases to conserve fat stores. Conversely, when your fat content rises above the set point, your body responds with a decrease in appetite and an increase in BMR. Hence, whether predestined as obese or lean, your body fights to maintain its fat content within preset limits.

5. *The wrong solution.* These problems notwithstanding, some people can't keep excess

weight off because of a more basic reason: Dieting does not attack the real cause of obesity. While most of the population attributes obesity to overeating, there is clear evidence to the contrary. In an article on successful weight-loss programs, Dr. Peter Wood indicates that Americans have become fatter in the past sixty years while per capita food consumption has *decreased*. Even on an individual basis, several research studies (e.g., survey of 1,485 London civil servants) have shown that food intake decreases with increasing fatness.

Thus, it appears that overeating cannot be the cause of obesity, nor can dieting be the correct remedy. What then?

MOVING MORE

As you may have guessed already, fat accumulates not so much from overeating as from underdoing. For example, obese people have been found to spend up to four times as many hours watching television as do thin people. And fat people walk an average of 2.2 miles a day, whereas a normal-weight person walks about 4.8 miles a day.[6]

Why is an increase in physical activity so much more effective than dieting for weight loss? First, an increased number of calories are burned during the activity. While some people argue that it takes a great deal of effort (e.g., walking thirty-five miles) to lose one pound of fat, they completely ignore the cumulative effects of activities. (One half hour of daily walking produces a fat loss of fifteen to twenty pounds per year.)

Second, after vigorous activity, the metabolic rate usually remains elevated for several hours, thereby burning even more calories than at normal, sedentary levels.

Third, participation in regular exercise often is accompanied by an increase in the basal metabolic rate, again cummulatively burning more calories than at sedentary levels. This increase in BMR may result from, among other factors, the significant increase in muscle mass that generally accompanies an exercise program.

A fourth and final influence of physical activity upon fat content involves the set point theory. Exercise appears to be the only effective and healthy way to lower the preset level of fat that the body strives to maintain. Thus, the overall effect of this increase in physical activity is a significant increase in energy production (calorie-burning), a significant increase in lean body tissue (better shape and tone), and a significant decrease in fat content. By comparison, dieting sadly promises decreased levels of energy production, no change or a decrease in lean body tissue, and no permanent change in fat content.

WALKING, GOD'S PERFECT EXERCISE
If you have a weight or fat problem, the best exercise to help you control your body weight is walking. It is pleasurable, safe, and convenient. In addition, walking is for anyone,

it's aerobic — which means it's good for your heart — and it fits your life-style. It's also a great family activity.

To get started on walking, do the following:

Week 1: Walk 10 to 15 minutes — nonstop. Don't worry about speed; walk at a pace that feels good to you. Do this four times this week.

Week 2: Walk 15 to 20 minutes four times this week. Follow the same guidelines as for week 1.

Week 3: Walk 20 to 25 minutes four times this week. Follow the above guidelines.

Week 4: Walk 25 to 30 minutes four times this week. Follow the above guidelines.

Week 5 & 6: Walk 30 minutes four times each week. Follow the above guidelines.

Walking the number of minutes at the designated heart rate on Table 10 will cause you to use about 300 calories.

Follow this walking regiment for at least four weeks. After that time, you may find you need to walk farther or faster because you are getting in better shape and your heart rate range may have increased.

OTHER EXERCISES

When your body and head call out for more or different exercise, consider these exercises:

Aerobics. Advantages: A fun activity for all ages and both sexes.

Disadvantages: You cannot know if you improve from week to week, other than by subjective feelings. Also, aerobics has a fairly high

TABLE 10

**NUMBER OF MINUTES OF RECOM-
MENDED WALKING AT DIFFERENT TRAIN-
ING HEART RATES**

Percentage of Maximum Heart Rate	Number of Minutes to Walk
40%	65:01–72:00
45%	57:31–65:00
50%	50:01–57:30
55%	42:31–50:00
60%	35:01–42:30
65%	30:01–35:00
70%	20:01–30:00

injury rate, especially among older women who try to do too much too soon.

Calories: Uses 4 to 10 calories a minute.

Bicycling and Stationary Bicycling. Advantages: Bicycling is an excellent fat-control activity for practically all ages. It can provide you with a vigorous workout. It not only strengthens the leg muscles but also subjects the body to little wear and tear.

Disadvantages: Most people pedal too slowly to derive the full fat-burning benefit. Cycling at eight miles per hour will not, as a rule, burn a significant number of calories. If you are relying on bicycling as a primary fat-burning exercise, pedal fast, ride up hills, and/or use a gear that offers substantial resistance.

Calories: Uses 3 to 10 calories a minute.

Cross-Country Skiing. Advantages: It burns more calories than any other fat-burning exercise.

Disadvantages: You can't ski year-round. In some parts of the country, you can't ski at all.

Calories: Uses 4 to 12 calories a minute.

Running. Advantages: Running is an excellent activity for reducing body fat.

Disadvantages: Running is not for everyone. It can shorten the muscles in the back of your legs, reduce flexibility, and make you prone to injury and leg pain. Obese people may find it too hard on their legs, knees, and ankles.

Calories: Uses 5 to 10 calories a minute.

Running-in-Place and Rope-Jumping. Advantages: These activities are good rainy-day replacements for outdoor activities.

Disadvantages: Most people who rope-jump or run-in-place find that motivation is the basic problem. These activities tend to cause knee and ankle pain. It also is difficult to measure progress.

Calories: Both use 4 to 10 calories a minute.

Stair Climbing. Advantages: This activity burns a lot of calories.

Disadvantages: Extremely boring. It may be too demanding for most people and is suggested only as a supplement to another activity.

Calories: Uses 7 to 15 calories a minute.

Swimming. Advantages: An extremely effective activity for the obese. The water provides support, so swimmers have fewer problems with their ankles, knees, and hips.

Disadvantages: You need a pool and the ability to swim. You also may find it hard to keep going for an extended period of time. When you become an extremely efficient swimmer, you may have difficulty burning enough calories.

Calories: Uses 5 to 10 calories a minute.

In addition to the walking program and other exercises, it's good simply to move more. Learn to do things the hard way:

- Park your car in the farthest parking spot.
- Walk to the store when possible.
- Get off public transportation two or three blocks from your destination.
- Use the stairs, rather than the escalator or elevator.
- Move as much as possible.

These kinds of activities can help you burn off an extra 25 to 100 calories a day—or 2.5 to 10 pounds a year.

EATING LESS AND MOVING MORE

The best way to lose weight and fat is to exercise, but this method may be too slow for some people. As a result, I propose a slight reduction in calories and an increase in activity. Most people can cut 100 to 200 calories a day without excessive hunger—but don't cut more than that.

Here are the foods to eat less of. They are high-calorie and low-nutrition. The foods are listed with the calories per item and the amount that gives you 200 calories. Each day eliminate one or several of these foods to reduce your calorie intake by 200 calories.

Now you know how to lose weight. This type of approach—eating less and moving more—has several advantages:

1. You'll lose fat and weight.

2. It is not difficult; most of us can part with 200 calories a day.

3. Since you're exercising, you'll get fit as you lose weight.

4. The life-style adjustments you need to make are small. That's the best way to make changes. Mark Twain said, "Habit is habit and not to be flung out the window by any man [or woman], but coaxed down the stairs one step at a time." That's good advice on eating and exercising habits.

5. The weight-loss rate is reasonable – not too slow, not too fast. You lose about a pound a week.

FAMILY WEIGHT CONTROL ACTIVITIES
● Trigger Stories

The purpose of these stories is to help children and adults understand the feelings of an overweight person. Present them after a meal, when driving in a car, or during other family times together.

a. Bill, the New Boy (Ages 5–14)

Bill is new on the block. He is heavy and cannot play sports well. Your friends decide to stand in front of his window and call him "fatty." What could you do? What might happen?

b. Chocolate Chip Cookies (Ages 9–16)

Your father comes into your room just as you polish off a bag of chocolate chip cookies. He says, "For the last time, cut it out. You have to make up your mind to stop overeating. Have some willpower. It's just a matter of disciplining yourself. If you don't, you'll end up fat like all your friends." How do you feel? What can you say?

c. Mary (Ages 10–16)

Mary, a teenager, has about ten pounds to lose and worries about the extra weight. One evening she was at a party and overate. Later that night she was so mad at herself for eating so much, she went outside and forced herself to vomit. She felt better because she knew the food was out of her system. How do you feel about Mary's behavior?

d. Tummy Flattener (Ages 8–16)

Businessman John Smith looks very important in his suit. He is careful to buy clothes that fit him well and make him look trim. He also makes sure he always is tan. If John gains extra weight, he starves himself until he loses it. Lately he's had trouble keeping his weight down, so he is wearing a tummy flattener under his shirt. As long as he looks good, he feels good. What do you think?

e. Sensitive Joan (Ages 8–16)

Joan is quite overweight. So are her parents and all of her grandparents. Joan watches what she eats, plays sports, and is quite active, but still struggles with her weight. She gets teased a lot because she is so heavy, and the boys don't ask her out on dates. Joan is very nice though. She is sensitive, caring, and loyal to her friends. How do you think you could help Joan feel better about herself?

● You and Your Friends' Eating Habits (Ages 12–16)
If you agree with the statement below, circle the letter *T*. If not, circle the letter *F*.

T   F   a.   My friends and I rarely eat breakfast.

T   F   b.   When we do eat breakfast, it tends to be coffee, sweet rolls or donuts, rather than a blend of cereal, milk, fruit and toast.

T   F   c.   My friends and I tend to eat quite a bit of low-nutrition/high-calorie convenience foods.

T   F   d.   Between meals most of us eat high-calorie/high-sugar snacks, rather than fruits and vegetables.

T   F   e.   My friends and I drink two or more colas or sodas a day.

T   F   f.   My friends and I tend to be very casual about the types of food we eat.

T   F   g.   Our place of employment or school does not serve nutritious meals. When it does, the foods generally are extremely high in calories.

T   F   h.   My friends and I are meat and potato eaters. We eat few fruits, vegetables, and salads, but a lot of animal protein.

T F i. My friends and I tend to select restaurants based on the quantity, rather than quality, of food. (Quality refers to a wide selection of foods, prepared nutritiously and relatively low in fat, salt, sugar, and caffeine.)

After taking this brief test, review your answers carefully. If you circled three or more *Ts*, you can conclude that your environment and friends encourage you to eat the wrong kinds of food. If that is the case, plan some ways to change this today. Record your observations and explain them to the rest of the family.

● Diary (Ages 8–16)
If you or your child want to change or add a behavior, keep track of it by making a diary. Fill a small notebook with pages like those on pages 92 and 93 of this book, or adapt these charts for your chosen behavior. Carry your diary with you at all times.

If you want to control the food that you eat, record in your diary everything you put into your mouth—water, pie, cake, bean sprouts, carrots, cake batter, pencils—everything. Include the time, place, your feelings, and, if possible, the calories, or at least the portion size. Or use your diary to monitor your feelings of stress (when you experience it, when you don't); your exercise level (everything from sleeping to running); drug usage; or any other behavior.

Why is a diary useful? (1) It shows you problem patterns and habits. You will be amazed at what you will learn about yourself. (2) Keeping a diary probably will change your habits. You will be more conscious of what you are doing, so you probably will tend to do some things less and others more. You might hesitate to reach for a bag of M & M's or be more prone to go for a walk. (3) It allows you to compare your current behavior with what you did several weeks ago. (4) It acts as an incentive.

At the end of each week, you may want to plot changes that you've noticed. This might include, "I'm eating less food between meals, I'm drinking less soda pop, I'm eating fewer desserts." Your evaluation can be subjective and objective.

Instructions for Using Your Food Diary
1. Complete the diary right after eating.
2. Note the time when you started eating.
3. Note where you were eating.
4. Note what you were doing while eating (e.g., reading, cooking, watching television).
5. Fill in the food and the amount.
6. Look up and enter the number of calories in each food.

Instructions for Using Your Exercise Diary
1. On a scale from 1 to 5, record your preexercise attitude level (1 being minimal stress, 5 being highly stressed).

2. Record pre-exercise heart rate, range of heart rate during exercise, and post-exercise recovery heart rate (taken one minute following exercise). The quicker the return of your pulse rate to normal — or to lower levels — the better the condition of your heart.

3. On a scale from 1 to 5, record your attitude regarding the outcome of your workout (1 being poor, 5 being great).

FOOD DIARY

Day: _____ Date: _____

Time	Where You Were	Activity	Your Feelings	Food and Amount	Calories
6:00 A.M.–11:00 A.M.					
11:00 A.M.–4:00 P.M.					
4:00 P.M.–9:00 P.M.					
9:00 P.M.–6:00 A.M.					

EXERCISE DIARY

Date: _____

	M	T	W	Th	F	S	S
Number of Hours of Sleep Night Before							
Pre-Exercise Attitude							
Activity							
Time of Day							
Length of Workout							
Heart Rates: Pre-, During, Post-							
Post-Exercise Attitude							

Weight: _____

TABLE 11

HIGH-CALORIE/LOW-NUTRIENT FOODS

Food	Calories Per Item	200-Calorie Amount
Vegetables		
French fries	17 each	12 average
Pickles, dill or sour	15 each	13 large
Pickles, sweet	25 each	8 small
Vegetables, canned	41/1½ cup	1½ cups
Salted vegetable juices	13/ounce	16 ounces
Fruit		
Peaches in syrup, canned	125 each	1½
Apricots, dried	32 each	6
Fruit drinks	19/ounce	10 ounces
Avocado	425	½
Sweetened fruit	250/cup	¾
Meat, Fish, Lentils, Nuts, and Eggs		
Visible fat, any meat	50/tsp.	4 tsp.
Bacon	33/strip	6 strips
Corned beef	62/ounce	3 ounces
Hot dogs	125 each	1½
Salami	125/ounce	1½ ounces
Luncheon meats	62/ounce	3 ounces
Duck/Goose	300/avg. serv.	⅔ serving
Sausages	250 each	¾
Patés	50/Tbsp.	¼ cup
Oily fish, such as:		
Herring, fresh	225/avg. serv.	9/10 serving
Mackerel, fresh	150/avg. serv.	1⅓ serving
Sardines, canned	25 each	8
Tuna, oil-pack	500/cup	3/8 cup
Deep-fried poultry	325/avg. serv.	3/5 serving
Spareribs	41 each	5 avg. ribs
Egg yolks	60 each	3⅓ average
Nuts	15 each	13
Beans, kidney/navy	200/cup	1 cup
Peanut butter	100/Tbsp.	2 Tbsp.
Shellfish:		
Crab, unshelled	30/ounce	6⅔ ounces
Shrimp, fresh	10 each	20 average
Thick stews	250/cup	¾ cup

Food	Calories Per Item	200-Calorie Amount
Grains, Breads, Cereals		
Presweetened cereal/granola	130/ounce	1½ ounce
Packaged cereals	110/ounce	1¾ ounce
Crackers, white	15/2" square	13 2" square
White bread	65/slice	3 slices
Muffins	125 each	1½
Oils and Fats		
Lard	125/Tbsp.	1½ Tbsp.
Butter/Margarine (regular)	100/Tbsp.	2 Tbsp.
Mayonnaise	100/Tbsp.	2 Tbsp.
Milk and Milk products		
Cream, 20%	33/Tbsp.	6 Tbsp.
Ice cream	150/scoop	1⅓ scoops
Ice milk	125/scoop	1½ scoops
Cream cheese	50/Tbsp.	4 Tbsp.
Sour cream	400/cup	½ cup
Cheeses (hard)	100/ounce	2 ounces
Whole milk/yogurt	167/cup	1¼ cups
Snack foods and Other		
Cake	125/1" slice	1½ slices
Pie	2800 each	1/8
Chocolate	50/Tbsp.	4 Tbsp.
Donuts, plain	150/avg. size	1⅓ average
Potato chips	200/cup	1 cup
Pretzels	16/avg. size	12½ avg.
Cookies	125/ounce	1½ ounces
Syrups	60/Tbsp.	3⅓ Tbsp.
Soda pop	12.5/ounce	17 ounces
Candy, small	50/bite size	4 bites
Animal crackers	8 each	25
Fig bars	50 each	4
Popcorn with butter & salt	65/cup	3 cups
Sherbet	100/scoop	2 scoops
Jam/Jelly	50/Tbsp.	4 Tbsp.
Pizza, mushroom	1200/medium	1/6 medium
Puddings	400/cup	½ cup

NOTES

CHAPTER 1
1. Jill Neimark, "Medical News," *American Health*, 3 (December 1984):14.
2. International Medical News Service, "Finds Children Are 'Enormously Competent at Self Care'," *Pediatric News* 18 (October 1984):67.
3. Louis Harris and Associates, Inc., *Prevention in America: Steps People Take—or Fail to Take—for Better Health*, in Charles T. Kuntzleman and Debra Drake, *The Feelin' Good Report* (Spring Arbor, Mich): Fitness Finders, 1984), 172-175.
4. Nedra Belloc and Lester Breslow, "Relationship of Physical Health Status and Health Practices," *Preventive Medicine* 1 (1972):409-421.
5. Alexander Comfort, *A Good Age* (New York: Crown Publishers, 1976) 140; Charles T. Kuntzleman, *Concepts for Wellness* (Spring Arbor, Mich.: Arbor Press, 1982), 175; and Pelletier, *Longevity*, 1-33.

CHAPTER 2
1. Kenneth H. Cooper, Michael L. Pollock, R. P. Martin, S. R. White, A. C. Linnerud, and A. Jackson, "Physical Fitness Levels versus Selected Coronary Risk Factors," *Journal of American Medical Association* 236 (12 July 1976), 166-169.
2. *Healthy People: The Surgeon General's Report on Health Promotion and Disease Prevention* (Washington, D.C.: U.S. Department of Health, Education and Welfare, 1979), 119-138.

3. Ibid.
4. Samuel M. Fox, "Relationship of Activity Habits to Coronary Heart Disease," in *Exercise Testing and Exercise Training in Coronary Heart Disease*, John P. Naughton and Herman K. Hellerstein, ed. (New York: Academic Press, 1973), 13.
5. Alexander Melleby, *The Y's Way to a Healthy Back* (New Jersey: New Century Publishers, Inc., 1982), 3.
6. Wendy Murphy and the Editors of Time-Life Books, *Dealing with Headaches* (Alexandria, Va.: Time-Life Books, 1982), 6-9.

CHAPTER 3

1. *Healthy People*, 60-67.
2. Jean Mayer, *Health* (New York: D. Van Nostrand, 1974), 135.
3. Gerald S. Berenson, *Cardiovascular Risk Factors in Children* (New York: Oxford University Press, 1980), 3-18.
4. Ibid., 3-18.
5. Richard Passwater, *Supernutrition* (New York: Dial Press, 1975), 19.
6. Sheryl London, *Anything Grows* (Emmaus, Penn.: Rodale Press, 1984).

CHAPTER 4

1. Steven Findlay, "Sowing the Seeds of Adulthood Disease," *USA Today* (7 March 1985), 4D.
2. Sally Ann Steward, "When Is Obesity a Burden to Health?" *USA Today* (12 February 1985), 4D.
3. Josh McDowell, *His Image . . . My Image* (San Bernardino, Calif.: Here's Life Publishers, 1984), 31.
4. Charles T. Kuntzleman, *Diet Free!* (Emmaus, Penn.: Rodale Press, 1982), 27.
5. W. Bennett and J. Gurin, "The New Set Point Theory," *The Dieter's Dilemma* (New York: Basic Books, 1982).
6. Frank I. Katch and William D. McArdle, *Nutrition, Weight Control, and Exercise*, 2nd ed. (Philadelphia: Lea and Febiger, 1983), 189.

About the Author

CHARLES T. KUNTZLEMAN is a professional health and fitness consultant to YMCAs, corporations, schools, health clubs, and individuals. He also serves as the national director for the Feelin' Good Program and is an adjunct professor of health services at Spring Arbor College. Among his sixty-plus books are *The No-Diet Fitness Book* and *The Well Family Book*. Dr. Kuntzleman lives in Spring Arbor, Michigan, with his wife, Beth. They have five children.

More Health Tips from Charles Kuntzleman

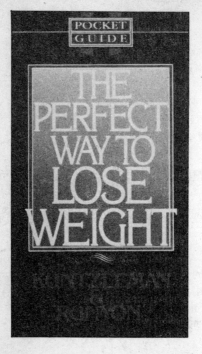

Available at your local Christian bookstore.

■ *Increase Your Personality Power* by Tim La-Haye. Why do you get angry? Afraid? Worried? Discover your unique personality type, then use it to live more effectively—at home, on the job, and under pressure. 72-1604-3 $2.25.

■ *Landing a Great Job* by Rodney S. Laughlin. Here are the essentials of a successful job hunt. Everything you need—from finding openings to closing interviews, and accepting offers. 72-2858-0 $2.25.

■ *The Perfect Way to Lose Weight* by Charles T. Kuntzleman and Daniel V. Runyon. Anyone can lose fat—and keep it off permanently. This tested program, developed by a leading physical fitness expert, shows how. 72-4935-9 $2.25.

■ *Strange Cults in America* by Bob Larson. An easy-reading update of six well-known cults: the Unification Church, Scientology, The Way International, Rajneesh, Children of God, and Transcendental Meditation. 72-6675-X $2.25.

■ *Surefire Ways to Beat Stress* by Don Osgood. A thought-provoking plan to help rid your life of unhealthy stress. Now you can tackle stress at its source—and win. 72-6693-8 $2.25.

■ *Temper Your Child's Tantrums* by Dr. James Dobson. You don't need to feel frustrated as a parent. The celebrated author and "Focus on the Family" radio host wants to give you the keys to firm, but loving, discipline in your home. 72-6994-5 $2.25.

■ *Terrific Tips for Parents* by Paul Lewis. The editor of *DADS ONLY* newsletter shares his findings on building character, confidence, and closeness at home. 72-7010-2 $2.25.

■ *When the Doctor Says, "It's Cancer"* by Mary Beth Moster. Cancer will strike approximately three out of four American families. Find out how to cope when you or someone you love hears this diagnosis. 72-7981-9 $2.25.

■ *When Your Friend Needs You* by Paul Welter. Do you know what to say when a friend comes to you for help? Here's how to express your care in an effective way. 72-7998-3 $2.25.

The books listed are available at your bookstore. If unavailable, send check with order to cover retail price plus $.50 per book for postage and handling to:

Christian Book Service
Box 80
Wheaton, Illinois 60189

Prices and availability subject to change without notice. Allow 4-6 weeks for delivery.